Interview with Jeffery Khoury, Bringing Telemedicine to the People

An Entrepreneur Revolutionizing Telemedicine with the Doctor Pocket™ Application

Richard G Lowe, Jr

Interview with Jeffery Khoury, Bringing Telemedicine to the People

An Entrepreneur Revolutionizing Telemedicine with the Doctor Pocket™ Application

Interviews with Influencers Series #2

Published by The Writing King
www.thewritingking.com

Interview with Jeffery Khoury, Bringing Telemedicine to the People

ASIN: B01GBC71J8
ISBN: 978-1-943517-89-3(Hardcover)
ISBN: 978-1-943517-27-5 (Paperback)
ISBN: 978-1-943517-28-2 (eBook)

Dedication

Forever grateful for the support of family and friends.

Table of Contents

A Special Note about how this book was created

Dear reader,

Thank you for buying your copy of *Interview with Jeffery Khoury Bringing Telemedicine to the People*.

This book explains the background of the Doctor Pocket application and its entrepreneur creator Jeffery Khoury.

This book was transcribed from a live interview.

That's why it reads as a conversation rather than a traditional "book" that talks "at" you.

Sincerely,

Jeffery Khoury

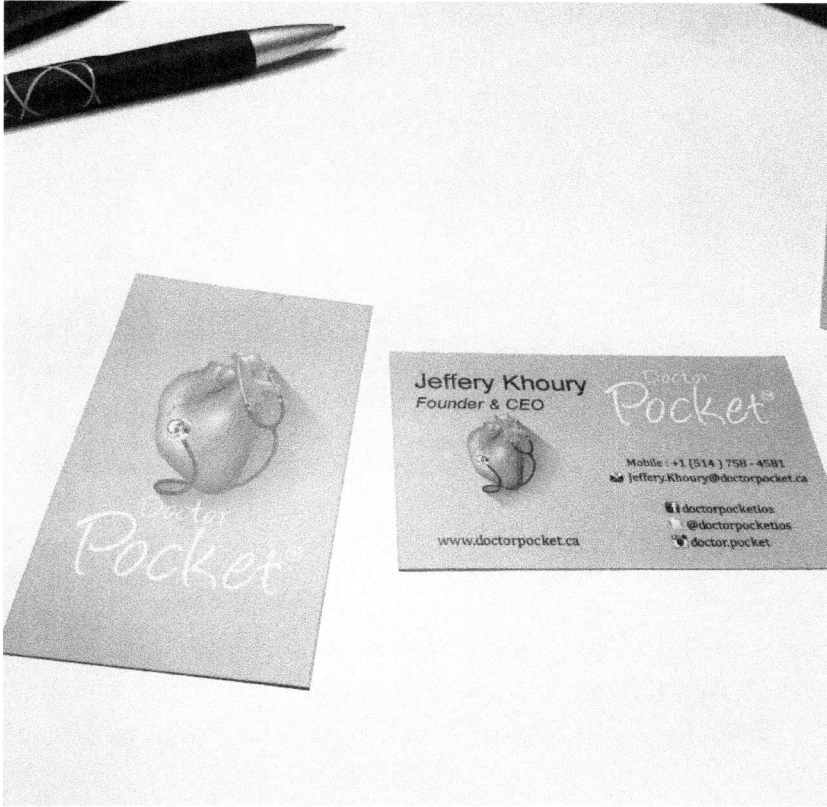

Interview

Richard Lowes (RL): Could you tell us a little bit about yourself in terms of your background, education and experience?

Jeffery Khoury (JK): Of course. I'm a 20-year-old full time student studying at John Molson School of Business (JMSB). I am in my first year of Finance.I was born and raised in Montreal, went to kindergarten, elementary and high school there.

However, my year abroad was probably the most important part of my college career—the year that really shaped me as a person. That experience opened up my eyes to a different world.

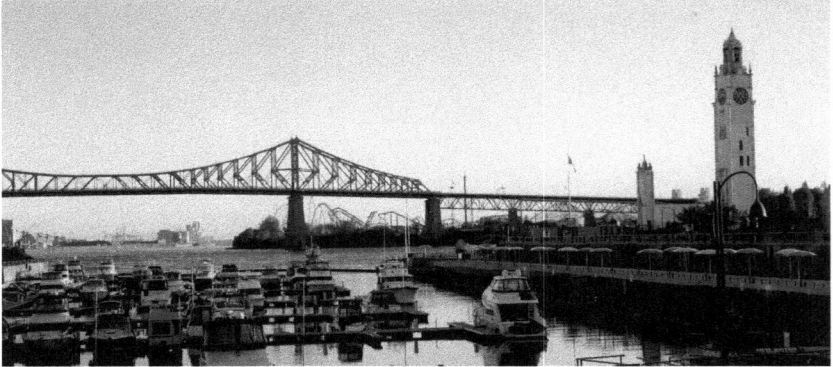

RL: What kind of an experience was that?

JK: In grade twelve I met a bunch of people that helped to broaden my knowledge about the world, and from those people I learned that life isn't simmering just in Montreal. I was born here, raised here, studied here, so for me, everything was based in Canada.

It was an interesting and enriching experience to travel abroad and also learn great values. I learned to value my family in a way I had never done before. It was definitely a necessary and important eye-opener.

RL: Could you go into more details about the morals and family values that you learned?

JK: Morals and family values—in North America every minute is calculated, the day passes by so quickly, the week passes by even faster. You have back to back meetings and less time to spend with the family.

I learned abroad that you have a day where you spend it solely with your family, then you have your time for your friends and time for your studies. But out of all of them, connecting and bonding with your family is a priority. The way people value their life is by focusing on the quality, not the quantity, by making everything so relaxed.

In North America, everyone is running around, and it's really hard to find time for your family—it opened my eyes to see how much time we really have and how we could use it to sit down not just with our friends but with our families too.

RL: And how did that make a difference in your life?

JK: It made a difference when I got ill. When I was abroad I got a bit sick, nothing serious, just a cold. But it was a cold that wouldn't go away.

I visited many doctors but no one was really helping me out. They were just giving me vitamins and over-the-counter medications. They prescribed me the basic cold treatment: rest more, take all your vitamins, drink lots of fluids. Even though I did all of those things, the cold still wouldn't go away.

That's when I got in touch with my cousin. He's a medical doctor, studying in New York right now. I asked him everything I had already asked the doctors.

"This is what's happening to me. I went to this doctor and I told him this, this and this. They gave me this vitamin to take. It's been 2- 3 weeks, and I still feel like I have my cold, what should I do?"

Because I was spending much more time talking to my family about my illness and not to the doctors within the country, I ended up thinking of ways I could improve the healthcare industry. Thanks to that cold I came up with an idea.

RL: What idea was that?

JK: *Doctor Pocket.* The telemedicine application I am launching allows you to speak with a real medical doctor rather than going simply through a Google search and getting frightened by other people's situations that you believe are similar to your own. But with *Doctor Pocket*, you will get the right answer for your specific condition by a doctor of your own choosing. With *Doctor Pocket* you're really getting tailored with the medical advice.

All the doctors I went to abroad couldn't really help me because I didn't feel that peace of mind I felt back home with a North American doctor.

So, through contacting my cousin, feeling that peace of mind every time we would talk and seeing the progress in my own health through his advice, I felt that everyone should be able to feel like they have a doctor in their pocket.

I saw the exponential demand and growth in the telemedicine industry and analyzed what's missing.

After seeing what is being done out there, the big names, how much demand there is for such an industry, I came up with my own unique approach for service, different than those currently out there.

RL: Could you give us an overview of telemedicine?

JK: Telemedicine is the communication between a doctor and a patient over the phone—a virtual consult. It could be done through a video call or a phone call. It's basically any practice of medicine that takes place when both parties are not physically in the same room.

RL: And how does it work?

JK: A good example of how it works would be describing the services of the major industry player *Doctor On Demand*. The way *Doctor On Demand* works is that you go into their application as a patient, you fill out a form, you tell them what's wrong with you, how long you've been feeling in a certain way, and what you've been feeling so to just to brief the medical professional.

After filling this form, they send it out to every single doctor on their platform and the first one that's available grabs it. After that you pay for the virtual consult with a doctor, prior to the physical consult.

How telemedicine works on the major player's application is that after you fill out a form you're instantly talking to a medical doctor that has the rundown of your situation. And on a 15-20 minutes video consult they tell you their opinion, so it's as if you're going into the doctor's clinic but instead of actually going there it's all happening on your phone. They could be half way around the world or down the block.

RL: Do you get a choice of doctor in those applications?

JK: No. Actually, regarding *Doctor On Demand*, the way it's being done is that right after you fill out your application, right off the bat, it's sent to every single doctor in their network so it's really up to who's available at that particular moment.

There are many other applications in which you don't have the chance to select the doctor you're talking to. Only once you talk to them do you see who they are and what type of specialty they're in. And that's when I realized the first major flaw with the current telemedicine industry: not having the freedom of choosing the MD for your own case.

RL: Do you think the inability to choose your doctor is appropriate?

JK: In my opinion: not at all. I knew there had to be a better way, and that's when *Doctor Pocket* came in.

I checked out the telemedicine industry, and it's a very booming industry. A lot of demand is there. I studied, analyzed and even experienced it myself to see what all the players are doing.

Because of all their exponential growth, the main players left a lot of voids in their market and one of the most important ones would be the interpersonal connection between the doctor and the patient pre- and post-virtual consult. That's how we, at *Doctor Pocket*, wanted to make a difference. The way we are making that difference is, essentially, by letting the users select what doctors they want to talk to and facilitate for them to follow-up with the same doctor they talked to in the first instance.

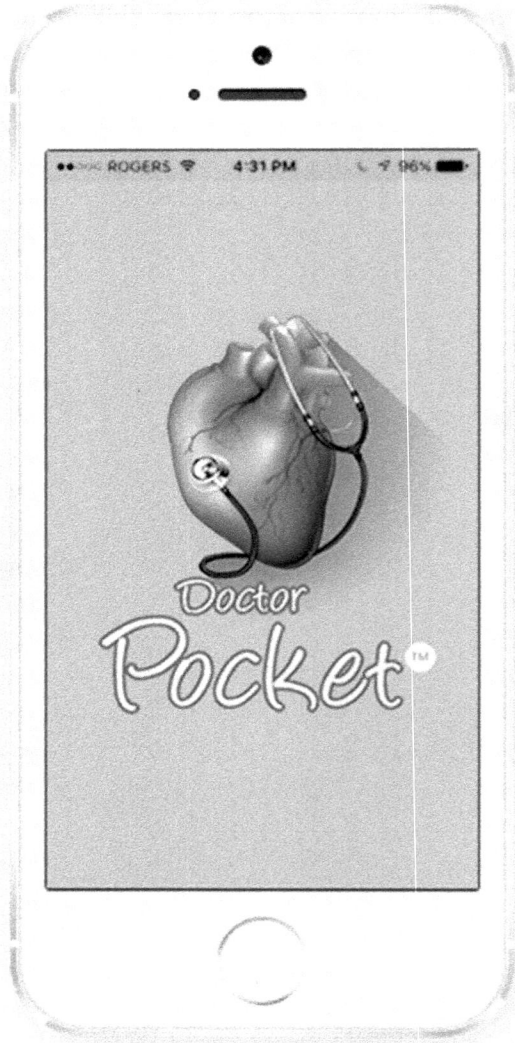

RL: So the users could choose the same doctor over and over again?

JK: Exactly. With Doctor Pocket Not only can the users choose the same doctor over and over again, but they can also choose who the doctors are before they even take their case to them. Users have access to the doctors' full profiles, they see where they're practicing, what kind of specialists they are; they have a link to their respective board certified profiles, they have brief bios on them. So, the users do not only choose who they talk to, but they also know who they talk to before they even call them.

RL: What kind of doctors do you have in your network?

JK: For the launch we are going to have around 25 to 30 doctors. Around a quarter of them are from the Ivy League schools such as Harvard Medical School, Stanford, Yale and also McGill.

Another major difference is that our network of doctors consists mostly of specialists. All the other competitors have General Practitioners as their MDs.

RL: You expect that to grow down the road?

JK: Of course. I find it a priority to hand-pick the doctors that we have on-board now since they will be the core reputation of our brand—think of it this way: when going to a restaurant that has an 18 to 20 page menu, no one is going to look through every single page, but when going to a high-class restaurant you usually have a one page menu, only of the chef's specials.

I really want to offer the entire world a list of the most credible and the most successful doctors, especially those that come from the Ivy League schools. The type of doctor that has the next

6 months booked at their private clinic but who can be reached through *Doctor Pocket* in minutes.

In addition to this, our medical team consists mostly of high-profiles doctors such as the Medical Director of Microsoft, the Medical Director of Walt Disney, Toyota America, BMW, United Airlines and even one of Ferrari's previous orthopedists.

RL: You're going to start out in the United States and Canada and then go out into the rest of the world?

JK: No, our launch is going to be International on a global scale. We have around 15 ambassadors worldwide. Our business team is currently present in Europe, Africa, China, around the United States, and, of course, Canada too.

Our ambassadors play an important role when the application is launched they let their communities know that the most efficient way to get connected to a doctor is through *Doctor Pocket.* Since the demand for Telemedicine is always going to be there—it's the healthcare industry, at the end of the day everyone is going to need to talk to a doctor at a certain point in their lives—our ambassadors will ensure proper coverage in their regions.

"I believe that everyone—despite their geographic location should take comfort in knowing they have a Doctor in their Pocket." Everyone should be entitled to an equal opportunity to connect with our greatly experienced and highly regarded Medical Doctors on-board; MDs from reputable Medical Schools such as Harvard, Stanford, Yale, Oxford, McGill, and many others. Having a specialist who is easily available and accessible—a *Doctor* in your *Pocket*, who can provide patients with valuable advice, who would always listen to you—can really make a huge difference."

RL: Is there a delay between signing up on the app and getting a doctor?

JK: Doctor Pocket offers a virtual platform where patients can interact with doctors. It's not an instant virtual consult because patients are able to choose which doctor to consult and their time of preference for when the appointment will take place. Once you make a request, the doctor you choose is notified about your request and if he is available for that 20-minute time frame consult—you'll get notified, and the time you chose, the date you chose, is when you're going to be speaking to them.

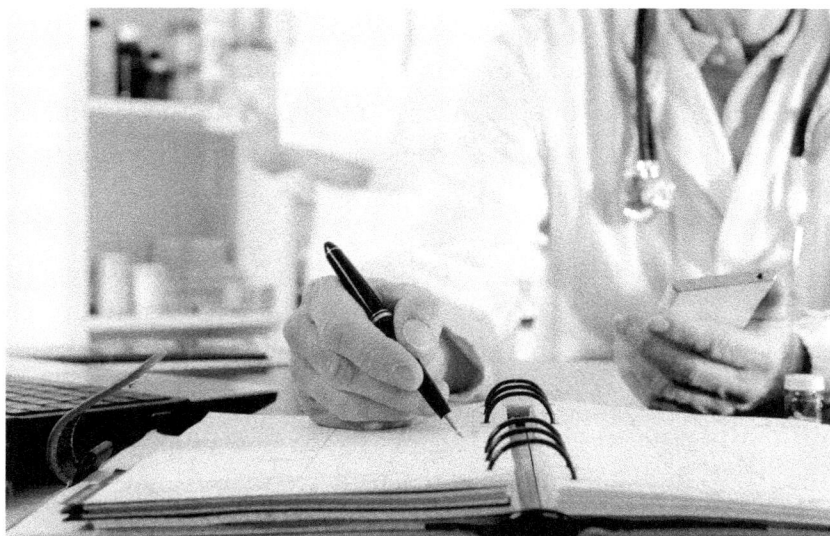

RL: Why would a physician want to get involved in the *Doctor Pocket* application?

JK: We allow the doctors to have a flexible work schedule. Doctors choose their rate for the 20-minute consult and how many hours they work. There are other telemedicine services available but this is what differentiates us.

The doctors who join us gain a unique opportunity to widen their network on a global scale. They can really make a difference because with Doctor Pocket they can offer their medical support to people around the globe , especially those in third world countries,. The doctors see many benefits in joining our team the biggest being convenience and working at their own schedule.

RL: What kind of medical advice could a patient get?

JK: Since we are the first telemedicine application doing this on a global scale, we have a lot of legal limitations, so it wouldn't be possible for a patient to consult with one of our doctors regarding a mental health case; if they're feeling unstable, any psychologist or psychiatrist consult would not be able to be done for our launch.

With that being said—we give the users a list of situations that they can bring to our doctors. Since, at the end of the day, the doctor and the patient aren't physically in the same room together, there are obviously going to be some limitations. **All that is drawn out clearly for the users of what we can help them with, what we can't in the app.**

The list containing the situations our doctors cannot consult them in is chronic conditions, mental health cases, cancer consults and those situations that our doctors would not feel comfortable to give advice to unless they are in physical contact with the patient.

RL: Could you give examples of what a patient could talk to the doctor about?

JK: They can contact the doctor for coughs, colds, allergies, sore throats, basically those symptoms, runny noses, swollen eyes, and second opinions on any sort of consults.

If a patient is going on a trip and wants to get connected to a doctor back home they can choose our doctors based on location, or if they want some sort of preventive and educational medicine for newborn babies, they could talk to our doctors for that too.

RL: Can they give advice based on medical tests?

JK: Of course, medical tests, they can look at scans such as X-Ray, CT scans, MRI. They could also look at blood tests too, all types of tests that could be electronically transferred in DICOM for scans or tests, for blood tests, that have the metrics that could be electronically transferred to our medical professionals that could be handled over the application too.

RL: What is a DICOM format?

JK: A DICOM format is basically the format that the radiologist gives you after scan to have that copy of your scan, be it MRI, CT scan or just a regular X-Ray.

RL: So, if a patient had had a tummy ache, he'd have to go to a local doctor first to get, say a CT scan, and then he can send that

CT scan to a doctor of his choice at *Doctor Pocket*'s to have him review it?

JK: Right, or if the patient is either exaggerating or even mitigating the situation our doctor could help them out with that.

Sometimes patients go to "Dr. Google" and try to diagnose themselves. They scare themselves into thinking they really need to go see a doctor because they've been feeling something that's irrelevant to whatever situation they are reading about. Our doctors could help them filter out the times they need to go in to see a doctor physically and get it checked out, or they are just exaggerating with a problem they think they have because of the web information. Many doctors have reported that it is very common for people to get imaginary or exaggerated illnesses based on what they read on the web.

RL: Can one of the doctors order a medical test for one of the patients somewhere else? So, if a patient called in with a bad back could the doctor then order the labs for that patient?

JK: Ok, that's actually a really interesting question. We're partnering up with a world-renowned hospital; it's one of the biggest hospitals and has an immense international presence. They have around 39 branches in France and what we are working out with them is exactly what you just said.

We will be offering them doctors on our application that can be reached for a virtual consult but we're also working with the hospitals on offering the patients all those machines the hospitals have that are free because of cancelled appointments or all those tests that can be done. Through *Doctor Pocket* the hospital is going to post their openings for people to come in person. Users could then book the time to take the test over the app. Once it is booked they could head to the hospital and the hospital would then instantly send the test to the doctor in charge of that particular case.

RL: And you'll be working on that in other countries as well in the future?

JK: Exactly. And the reason why I was interested in partnering up with this hospital is because they have a great international presence. They have hospitals all over the world, averaging 300 to 400 European Board Certified medical doctors. I thought that this would be a great place to start.

RL: That brings up another question. What about prescribing prescription drugs? Can a doctor do that?

JK: For the time being, since it's being done on a global scale, our doctors are staying away from any kind of prescription but our short-term goal would be to have a doctor in every region that a virtual consult is happening in.

The doctor that was located in your current region would either go over the consult with that medical professional that you've been talking to through the app or evaluate the user himself.

If you were in need of a prescription they would handle that locally. So, for the time being, it would not be possible until we had an MD representative in each region of the world we're offering virtual consults, something our ambassadors are in charge of.

RL: What if the patient calls in and the doctor realizes it's actually an urgent issue. Would s/he then order the patient to see an emergency room or urgent care?

JK: That's exactly it. If one of our doctors feels like the patient has been mitigating the situation and really taking it lightly, whenever it's something that really requires that in-person care, our doctors will tell the patient to go to the ER or go to a doctor as soon as possible.

RL: Let's get more into the application now from a patient point of view.

JK: From a patient point of view, it's an extremely simple and friendly user interface. What we wanted *Doctor Pocket* to do is to connect you with a specialist of your choice from the comfort of your own home or on the go.

What we really did is that we have our own encrypted platform, and this platform allows you to book and chat with any one of our specialists in real time.

On this platform you have text messages, voice notes, and multimedia. Our objective is for people all over the world to receive trustworthy information directly from our specialists

Something I've been imagining forever is a future where access to any physician is very quick, while avoiding exposure to infections from the clinic or the hospital. What *Doctor Pocket* is trying to do is connect that one and two.

The telemedicine industry is already out there, so what we are planning to do is to tackle it in a different way. What makes our approach so unique is that we modified and enhanced the interpersonal connection.

RL: I'm the user, I've got a head cold, I want to use *Doctor Pocket*, what do I do?

JK: As a user, you log into the app, you create your own account and with this account the most important thing that we need is your time zone since we're doing this on an international time zone configuration basis.

Whenever you're logged into the app you have your 4 icons: you have *you're about us*, **your share,** *how it works, and search doctor network.*

In the *about us* it tells you what we can help you with and what we can't help you with. In the *how it works* it tells you A to Z— everything about how the app is used and how to get started; you really just click *search network.* And in our network you can search doctors, you can scroll down the list and look at the doctor of your own choice or you could search doctor based on specialty, practice location or time zone availability.

After you search a doctor, you click his profile and once you click his profile you see everything about the doctor. After you have decided what doctor you want, you go ahead and you pick the date and time that you want to talk to them and you brief them about your situation. Boom, the virtual consult request is sent.

The doctor gets notified and sees: Patient X wants to talk to him or her on this date, at this time, for this reason, he accepts or reject appointment—the doctor accepts or rejects based on any criteria such as his own availability or the severity of the case.

If he accepts you get notified to pay the consultation fee.

After the confirmation from the doctor, all you're waiting for is your appointment time.

It all starts when you get notified that 'your appointment is now'.

It's a real time chatting platform with voice note and multimedia messages. You have the doctor at your disposal for 20 minutes and you can get the best advice out of it.

RL: Is this on a smart phone or is this on a computer?

JK: This is on a smart phone. Our iOS version is going to launch in around a month and our Android version is going to be launching in around 2-3 months. Our goal is to have *Doctor Pocket* on every smart phone.

RL: Do you have plans to put it on the desktop?

JK: As technology has been advancing and as people have been looking for the most efficient way out, I wanted this to be something that could be out of the comfort of your own home or on the go. So, I was focused more on, as people want the most efficient way out, having the doctor in their pocket, which is why I chose the name *Doctor Pocket*.

I'm not interested in having something that could be done on a desktop.

RL: How did you get the brainstorm of how to do this? How did that happen?

JK: How this happened is whenever I was abroad and I got sick I just wouldn't get better, I just didn't have that peace of mind with the local doctors.

Since most of my family members are medical doctors I would often reach out to my cousin and send him voice notes, pictures and basically just to ask him what's going on and get his opinion about it.

With my cousin I felt that peace of mind after sending messages back and forth through iMessage. So that's how the idea came to my mind. I talked to my mom about it and she thought it was a great idea that is worth pursuing.

It's great to be able to connect with a doctor or even a specialist at your fingertips instead of waiting 2-3 weeks or even 2-3 months to see a specialist.

RL: Now you thought of the idea, the next step is turning it into a product. So, could you tell me about that process?

JK: This is a funny story actually. I thought I could do it all by myself. I had the idea in mind, all I have to do is learn some basic app development and then it'll be complete.

I tried teaching myself coding; I tried teaching myself basically everything in app development, and it was something that was much harder than I had anticipated, something impossible for a business-oriented mind like mine. At that point I felt that it would take me years to complete everything I had in mind.

After that, I reached out to a development company. Their name is I-SOFTINC. They're the guys who made the closest location application for McDonalds and Applebee's.

They were already on the map doing applications for Fortune 500 companies so I gave them a call and I pitched them my idea and it developed into the app it is today.

Back then it was just connecting 1 and 2, and that's all I really cared about. Basically, with all the developers' expertise and their experts on-board we came up with a plan to take *Doctor Pocket* to where it's headed today.

Essentially, the first step to actually make it happen was to get the IT team done. And currently, today, our IT team is made up of around 10 people. They're developers, coders, designers, programmers, innovators, and people who work closely with Apple and Google Play regulations.

RL: Could you tell me how you put that team together?

JK: The IT team was put together through I-SOFTINC. I was talking to their CEO at first, and they guided me in terms of what I needed and who I needed on my team.

As the idea grew and as the features on the application grew, the IT team also grew with it. An example would be the international time zone configuration feature—it's something that no telemedicine service has out there.

What this feature really does is no matter where you are in the world or where our doctors are in the world we have a unique booking system to choose that doctor and be able to book him at whatever time it is and then block all those times out.

They developed a very advanced algorithm that basically allows anyone all over the world to be connected to all our doctors all over the world.

RL: You outsourced the development to this group?

JK: Yes, our developers are located in South-East Asia.

RL: What's the business model that you have for this?

JK: The current business model is this: our doctors are earning 60% of every virtual consult. For the potential users, we are starting *Doctor Pocket* as a free download.

The way the money gets involved is that after the user pays for the virtual consult. The split between the doctors and the company is 60/40. So, we have it on our website for any doctors that are interested in joining. They choose how much they work for. At the end of the month they get 60% of all the gross revenue that came in from their respective virtual consults.

RL: Now what role do the ambassadors play in this?

JK: The ambassadors are selected regional representatives whose communities would benefit greatly from this application. For example, the medical industry or the healthcare industry isn't advanced to the point where they could talk to such credible doctors. Sometimes the waiting time or expense is just way too much for the people to wait weeks to talk to a general practitioner or take a full day of work just from a simple cold. So what these ambassadors do is they let people in their region know that *Doctor Pocket* is the most efficient way of getting in contact with the most credible medical professionals of their choice at their convenience of time, **at the comfort of their homes.**

RL: So, the ambassadors are local advertisers and marketers?

JK: Exactly. They are local advertisers and marketers, and even more than that, they are the local footwork. They are the people who are going to make it happen in their region to really benefit their community—and the healthcare that their community is receiving.

RL: What was your biggest challenge that you had to overcome and how did you do it?

JK: I would say there were two. One of them being the development side and how many features we could begin with and the financial support. I overcame that through our sponsors *United Auto*. They have a dealership in Montreal. They also have an international brand too. Their racing team is based in Quebec.

Thanks to them, one of my first biggest challenges was now the last thing on my mind. Thanks to United Auto, we now have the funds we need for our development team to take us to the next level.

The second challenge was finding some high profile medical doctors, and reaching out to the Ivy League Med Schools. There were a lot of no's to get the 25-30 doctors we have on-board now. Some doctors were against telemedicine because it goes against their values they are not physically in the same room as the user.

I overcame this by not giving up. For every 1000 no's I would get 1 yes. We got a lot of yes's from very important people. Thankfully, a quarter of our medical team now are Harvard Medical School doctors.

Our greatest accomplishment would be the two high profiles we now have on-board. Number one would be Dr. Daniel Saurborn. He served as the Medical Director for Microsoft, Walt Disney, Toyota America and W America, and United Airlines.

He's a Harvard medical doctor. His specialty is radiology and he has a lot of experience in telemedicine. The reason why he went into medicine, actually, was because of telemedicine. He saw the value of how much he could help people over the phone, especially since he's a radiologist, so it's a very telemedicine friendly specialty as all their diagnostics are done based **on what they physically see.**

Having him on-board was one of my biggest accomplishments on the medical side, and an honor.

The second doctor would be Dr. Hazem Kobeissi, a German educated physician who specializes in orthopedic surgery. It was an honor to bring him on-board because he was part of the medical team traveling with Michael Schumacher.

Michael Schumacher is the retired seven-time formula world champion.

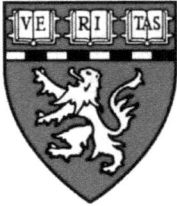

HARVARD
MEDICAL SCHOOL

Bringing both of these doctors on-board skyrocketed our credibility on the medical side. Once other medical doctors started seeing the Ivy League schools such as Harvard, Stanford, Yale and McGill, they became more open in joining our medical team.

Regarding the exposure, I had a Harvard Professor invite me to host a webinar for their medical students. This helped us in starting the buzz in the Ivy League Med Schools.

RL: Initially you had to explore getting the capital together to put this whole project together. What areas did you look for to get capital and how did you finally wind up at where you've wound up?

JK: The way *Doctor Pocket* began is thanks to the number one man I pitched my idea to— that man is my father. I would not be here at this position with a team over 50 without his ongoing advice and, of course, his seed investment.

I initially pitched him the idea after I got a quote from I-SOFTINC. I told him, "This is how much I need now; this is what I'm going to do and this is what I'm going to make happen."

He was happy about it. I got his 120% support wholeheartedly to get kick-started on my venture. Our interface was set up and everything was looking good, but it wasn't market ready yet.

To really take it to the next step is when we got interest from our sponsors: *United Auto*. And when they joined on-board it took *Doctor Pocket* to the next level.

We also have our ambassadors who invested to have royalty rights for their region.

RL: How are you promoting *Doctor Pocket* to doctors?

JK: At first it was all through my LinkedIn. I have around 14-15,000 followers and I started **with around 1,000 or 2,000**. Through my LinkedIn I was reaching out to high-profile doctors, pitching them my vision and my idea and seeing what they think.

Now I have alumni's from Harvard, alumni's from Stanford, alumni's from McGill that are going out and reaching out to the doctors themselves, and that's how we're getting our doctors on-board now. In the beginning, it was me going one-to-one, outlining the benefits to these doctors of what they would gain by joining *Doctor Pocket*.

RL: You have a team of people, these ambassadors and others who are going out to talk to doctors and finding out if they want to join?

JK: The ambassadors are there more to promote the product in the region, to get users but each ambassador sees the value of creating a network of doctors within their specific region.

The more doctors there are on *Doctor Pocket* in a certain region, the greater the probability that users would use it to get into contact with those doctors. But other than the ambassador's role, we have a doctor recruiter role and those are our well-connected doctors on-board. The doctor recruiters reach out to their network of doctors and get their colleagues interested and get them to join the team also.

RL: How does that work? Could you walk me through how a medical recruiter would get a doctor on-board?

JK: In the beginning, it was a long process. We had all the agreements that had to be signed. We gave our recruiters a doctor agreement and the limitations agreement of what they can say and what they can't say.

Then we need them to get all their basics which we would need– by basics I mean their name, their specialty, their practice location, a copy of their medical license and all these background checks had to be done through our recruiters, so it was a very long process to get a doctor to join the on-board team.

How it is now? It's very simple, very efficient, and goes hand in hand with the vision of *Doctor Pocket*—making everything as efficient as possible.

How we have it now is just through a simple link. So you go to *DoctorPocket.ca* and you just click on 'Join Our Medical Team' and through that the doctors apply to join. And when they apply they fill out all the basic information we need from them. They check off all the agreements we need from them and they've also attached a link of their profile on their respective boards and also an attachment of their medical licenses.

Now everything's done electronically. What all the medical recruiters—all the doctor recruiters—are doing is just sending out these links.

RL: Do the doctor recruiters just email links to doctors or they actually visit them in place and talk to them? How do they do this promotion?

JK: For the current doctor recruiters that we have on-board they are medical doctors themselves so they're constantly surrounded by other medical doctors in the environments that those doctors are joining.

How we have it now? The doctor recruiters just tell their colleagues what project they are part of, the vision of the project, and how these doctors could potentially help people like the current ones that are on-board, and through that, if some doctors are interested, just email them the link and through that link they have all the information available for them to see how it works, what they need in order to apply and what the benefits are for joining our team.

RL: How are you getting patients?

JK: Patients—we haven't gotten any yet since we're still at pre-launch phase. Our application is not on the app store yet. We're waiting on our Android version to be more developed, since I wanted to launch the iOS around mid-May and I wanted to launch the Android version around a month later.

We've had many people messaging us through our Facebook and Twitter pages for medical advice. Our social media presence has opened my eyes to how many people are in need to be connected to a doctor, how much demand there is to get in contact with a North American or European board certified specialist.

RL: Do you see yourself hiring, say, an advertising firm or something down the road to get it known to people?

JK: I think the best way to get this known to people would be through our medical team. I think that would be the best advertising ever to really show the people that the person on the other side is a certified specialist: high profile medical doctor that has not just experience in the medical industry but also has the experience in the telemedicine industry— a doctor that you would normally wait months to talk to.

RL: And how are you going to get the patients to know about it?

JK: Through our ambassadors—that's why I'm looking for ambassadors in certain regions of the world where I can't physically be in. Other than that I would say Facebook, Google ads, LinkedIn basic SEO and ASO. I believe social networking will be the best advertising channel for Doctor Pocket.

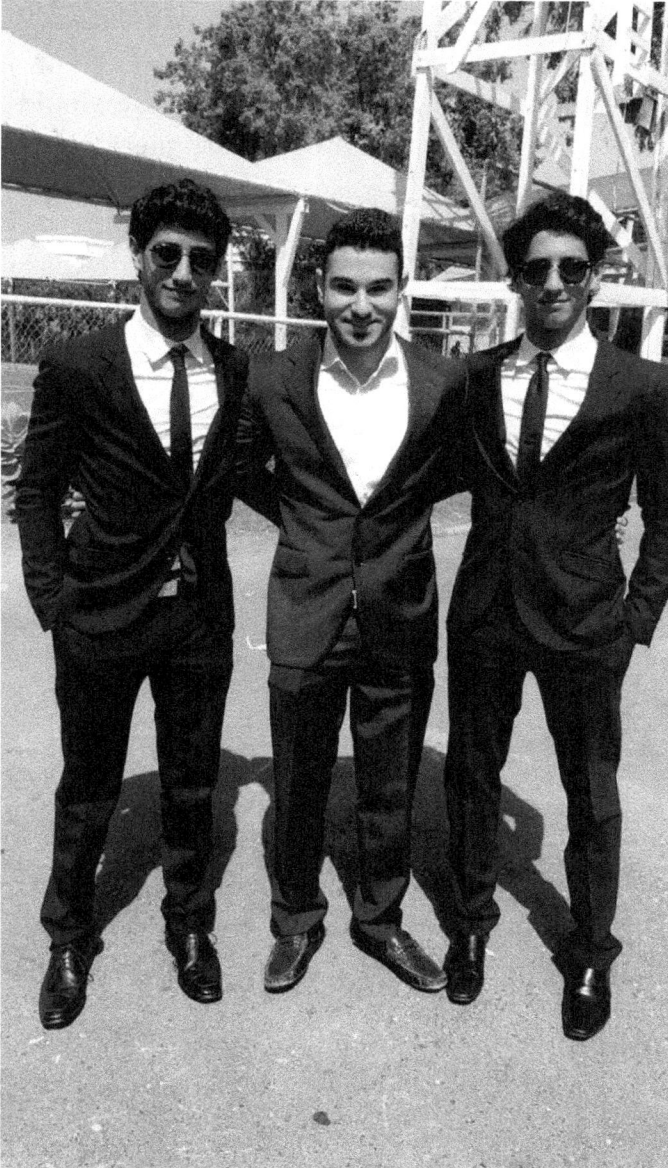

RL: What about television ads or things like that?

JK: I think the best thing instead of ads would really be, for example, an interview or a little talk about it; or just me physically being there. An example of that would be the opportunity I have to go speak to Harvard medical students in around 2-3 weeks.

One of their professors reached out to me; he teaches a health informational technology class and he liked the idea, liked the vision, and he reached out to me to see if I could come and introduce it to their students.

I think going to events like that, speaking at conferences, going to seminars would get us much better presence, attention and attraction rather than a TV ad. Something more informational than commercial would benefit *Doctor Pocket* the most.

RL: How does it feel to be an entrepreneur?

JK: Wow. It's an incredible feeling. I grow every single day. The motivation is something that's key to the success of an entrepreneur. I would say this project came about a year ago.

I thought I would be on the app store 7-8 months ago. That takes patience. I think learning how to be patient was kind of the hardest part for me of being an entrepreneur.

The best feeling is seeing all the support from other entrepreneurs out there that see the struggle, know the struggle and respect the motivation and the time and the dedication you have to put into an idea to make it a reality.

To be an entrepreneur, it's not a 9 to 5 job. It's something you lose sleep over, there have been countless times I've been eating a meal and I just randomly run to my basement and jot something down or run outside to take a call.

It's more of a lifestyle than a job, so, to be an entrepreneur it feels amazing because to be a good entrepreneur or, to be a *happy* entrepreneur I'd say, would be doing something that you're passionate about. I feel blessed to be working on what I'm passionate about. So, for me, to be an entrepreneur feels like a blessing.

RL: What advice would you give to people who want to be entrepreneurs?

JK: To really find something that they're most passionate about because to be an entrepreneur you need to be grinding 24/7, 365 days a year, always thinking about what you're working on.

Since you are passionate about what you are working on, your subconscious is going to be thinking about ways to grow, ways to get better.And, really, finding something that you're passionate about is going to make you go through that process of losing sleep, sacrificing your social life, stressing out about something that you want to do rather than need to do.

RL: What's the best part of being an entrepreneur?

JK: The best part would be to really see how far you can bring an idea. In no way did I ever think I could bring *Doctor Pocket* this far. To process that an idea that came to my mind would became an actual application—something that could actually help people, benefit people, potentially make a difference in the world—is probably the most amazing feeling.

Even though our product isn't live yet, we had around 18 consults already done. That is, those people that messaged me through Facebook who asked me some medical questions. I'm obviously not a medical doctor, but I get them in contact with the specific specialty that relates to their situations.

To see that these people that we already helped without even having an app out there–it just feels great. It feels really amazing to get the support from everyone that sees you working hard and it feels even greater to know that what you're working on will potentially make a difference in the medical world.

RL: For those budding entrepreneurs out there, what are some of the things that they should look out for?

JK: I would say that the biggest obstacle for any entrepreneur would be himself/herself. To look out for any limitations they set themselves because, literally, the sky is the limit as long as you believe in what you're doing and as long as you have the patience. Patience is the number one feature and attribute you need to have within or to learn how to build it gradually. Being impatient could really be the deal breaker in making your idea an actual product or just keeping it as, simply, an idea. To have patience and persistence in not limiting yourself would be the most important thing to focus on. Be Patient, Consistent, Persistent, Focused and have Self-Confidence shall help you great deal to overcome obstacles that you would encounter on your way.

RL: So, it's not the money, it's your own demons.

JK: It's your own demons. Essentially, the limits you set for yourself are real. During my adventurewith this project there's been a million, a million, a million times I could have said, "Ok, this is it." And I'm not the only one.

Every single entrepreneur that really started their own company or their own product, know that there are so many speed bumps along the way that you realize, "Wow, this is why people just keep these ideas and just give up half way."

Because,to really believe in yourself, to finish what you started——is the hardest part. The entrepreneurs should look out for not underestimating at all what their full potential really is.

RL: What do you recommend for them to do to overcome that?

JK: I'll recommend just being one with yourself. Giving yourself the time to pursue what you think is right instead of just letting the idea go.I say this because I've seen—I've heard many great ideas that just stayed as ideas because of the lack of persistence, motivation, passion, and most important–patience.

Something you really stick with and execute and make it happen could be the difference between an entrepreneur and just someone who has a good idea.

I have a really important understanding about the vision of *Doctor Pocket* and where I want to take it in the future.

RL: Why don't you talk about that?

JK: If anyone thinks to themselves what the limits are to telemedicine: the number one answer for the medical side and the potential patients would be the physical barrier.

The barrier for entry for many of the medical doctors that I wanted them to join on-board would be having that physical barrier. Telemedicine is a very controversial industry because of this very barrier.

What we're currently working on is completely removing the physical barrier of telemedicine.

The way we would do this would be integrating a medical device accessory to *Doctor Pocket*. The medical device industry is very advanced. There's a lot of advanced technology and products that's already out there.

The telemedicine industry is something that's currently booming so what I'm really focused on doing and what we're executing right now is linking both of those industries: the medical device industry and the telemedicine industry. Our goal is to have our MDs to be able to see the patient's vitals and even more through our medical wearable device.

This wearable medical device is going to calculate the heart-rate, blood pressure, body temperature, blood oxygen levels. We're even working on a patented technology that has an integrated microphone to hear heartbeat and lung functions.

That's our short term goal for connecting the medical device to the telemedicine application in order for our wearable device to *Doctor Pocket* would have the doctor see all the metrics, all the vitals, all the numbers you'd see if they were face-to-face with you in the same room even though they're half way across the world.

RL: Can you expand on that a little bit more? What do you see even beyond that?

JK: What I see beyond that is—our long term goal—to globalize our medical device so people could store their information, their patient history on our medical device and share it with our MDs on the application or even with a real life medical doctor.

By the wearable device, we're working on a bracelet that's going to link to our app via Bluetooth, and it's something that's really interesting because that technology is out there, but what we're creating is all in one device and using these metrics in a real-time virtual consult.

We're currently working on that right now. And I think that's what would put *Doctor Pocket* on the map and that's what would take telemedicine to the next level. To not limit the doctors to what the patient is telling them over the phone but really to give the doctors even more of what they would have if they were face to face with a patient even though they're really half way across the world.

RL: Are there any other questions that I didn't ask that you can answer?

JK: I would say the differentiation. I think, **I listed them already but all spread out**.

RL: Please go ahead and list them.

JK: Ok, I will list them concisely. Our differentiation on the user side is our user interface. Our user interface is very different. The way that it's different is that we include many configurations and many features that other telemedicine services don't have.

The number one thing would be an international time zone configuration. What this time zone configuration does is that we're basically the first telemedicine application to offer our medical services on a global scale.

With this time zone configuration, anyone, all over the world, could talk to anyone of our doctors on our unique appointment scheduling system. By the unique appointment scheduling system, essentially, it's us allowing our users to choose which doctor they would like to have a virtual consult with and at whatever time they wish on an international basis.

The third differentiation would be the interpersonal connection that I was emphasizing. This interpersonal connection occurs between all our medical doctors and users on *Doctor Pocket*. Each of them, the users and the medical doctors respectively have their own profiles, and on their profiles they have their profile pictures, their names. For the doctors—what they have is their practice locations, their gender, specialty and brief bios.

Another major difference would be the choice of communication channel. The major competitors force you to either text, which would be *Health Tap*, or video call, which would be *Doctors On Demand*.

On *Doctor Pocket* we offer the users the choice of whatever communication channel they would prefer. During a virtual consult you can either send the messages by text, voice note, video image, audio call, and video call. We've let the users choose the method of communication that they feel most comfortable with.

RL: Jeffery, thank you for a most fascinating interview. It was most enlightening.

JK: You're welcome. It was my pleasure. Thank you for the opportunity and for giving me the chance to tell the world about *Doctor Pocket*, how it began and where it's going.

Before you go

If you scroll to the last page in this eBook, you will have the opportunity to leave feedback and share the book with Before You Go. I'd be grateful if you turned to the last page and shared the book.

Also, if you have time, please leave a review on Amazon. Positive reviews are incredibly useful. If you didn't like the book, please email me at rich@thewritingking.com and I'd be happy to get your input.

About the Author

https://www.linkedin.com/in/richardlowejr
Feel free to send a connection request

Follow me on Twitter: @richardlowejr

Richard Lowe has leveraged more than 35 years of experience as a Senior Computer Manager and Designer at four companies into that of a bestselling author, blogger, ghostwriter, and public speaker. He has written hundreds of articles for blogs and ghostwritten more than a dozen books and has published manuscripts about computers, the Internet, surviving disasters, management, and human rights. He is currently working on a ten-volume science fiction series – the Peacekeeper Series – to be published at the rate of three volumes per year, beginning in 2016.

Richard started in the field of Information Technology, first as the Vice President of Consulting at Software Techniques, Inc. Because he craved action, after six years he moved on to work for two companies at the same time: he was the Vice President of Consulting at Beck Computer Systems and the Senior Designer at BIF Accutel. In January 1994, Richard found a home at Trader Joe's as the Director of Technical Services and Computer Operations. He remained with that incredible company for almost 20 years before taking an early retirement to begin a new life as a professional writer. He is currently the CEO of The Writing King, a company that provides all forms of writing services, the owner of The EBay King, and a Senior Branding Expert for LinkedIn Makeover. You can find a current list of all books on his Author Page and take a look at his exclusive line of coloring books at The Coloring King.

Richard has a quirky sense of humor and has found that life is full of joy and wonder. As he puts it, "This little ball of rock, mud, and water we call Earth is an incredible place, with many secrets to discover. Beings fill our corner of the universe, and some are happy, and others are sad, but each has their unique story to tell."

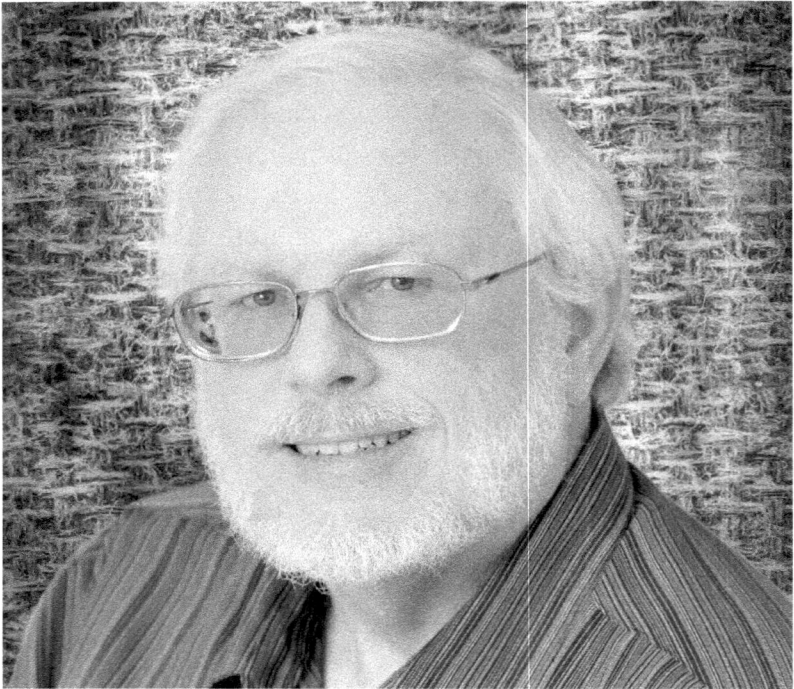

His philosophy is to take life with a light heart, and he approaches each day as a new source of happiness. Evil is ignored, discarded, or defeated; good is helped, enriched, and fulfilled. One of his primary interests is to educate people about their human rights and assist them to learn how to be happy in life.

Richard spent many happy days hiking in national parks, crawling over boulders, and peering at Indian pictographs. He toured the

Channel Islands off Santa Barbara and stared in fascination at wasps building their homes in Anza-Borrego. One of his joys is photography, and he has photographed more than 1,200 belly dancing events, as well as dozens of Renaissance fairs all over the country.

Because writing is his passion, Richard remains incredibly creative and prolific; each day he writes between 5,000 and 10,000 words, diligently using language to bring life to the world so that others may learn and be entertained.

Richard is the CEO of The Writing King, which specializes in fulfilling any writing need. You can find out more at https://www.thewritingking.com/, and emails are welcome at rich@thewritingking.com

Books by Richard G Lowe Jr.

Business Professional Series

On the Professional Code of Ethics and Business Conduct in the Workplace – Professional Ethics: 100 Tips to Improve Your Professional Life - have you ever wondered what it takes to be successful in the professional world? This book gives you some tips that will improve your job and your career.

Help! My Boss is Whacko! - How to Deal with a Hostile Work Environment - sometimes the problem is the boss. There are all kinds of managers, some competent, some incompetent, and others just plain whacked. This book will help you understand and handle those different types of managers.

Help! I've Lost My Job: Tips on What to do When You're Unexpectedly Unemployed – suddenly having to leave your job can be a harsh and emotional time in your life. Learn some of the things that you need to consider and handle if this happens to you.

Help! My Job Sucks Insider Tips on Making Your Job More Satisfying and Improving Your Career – sometimes conditions conspire to make the regular trek to a job feel like a trip through Dante's Inferno. Sometimes, these are out of our control, such as a malicious manager or incompetent colleague. On the other hand, we can take control of our lives and workplace and improve our situation. Get this book to learn what you can do when your job sucks.

How to Manage a Consulting Project: Make money, get your project done on time, and get referred again and again – I found that being a consultant is a great way to earn a living. Managing a consulting project can be a challenge. This book contains some tips to help you so you can deliver a better product or service to your customers.

How to be a Good Manager and Supervisor, and How to Delegate – Lessons Learned from the Trenches: Insider Secrets for Managers and Supervisors – I've been a manager for over thirty years I learned many things about how to get the job done and deliver quality service. The information in this book will help you manage your projects to a high level of quality.

Focus on LinkedIn – Learn how to create a LinkedIn profile and to network effectively using the #1 business social media site.

Home Computer Security Series

Safe Computing is Like Safe Sex: You have to practice it to avoid infection – Security expert and Computer Executive, Richard Lowe, presents the simple steps you can take to protect your computer, photos and information from evil doers and viruses. Using easy-to-understand examples and simple explanations, Lowe explains why hackers want your system, what they do with your information, and what you can do to keep them at bay. Lowe answers the question: how to you keep yourself say in the wild west of the internet.

Disaster Preparation and Survival Series

Real World Survival Tips and Survival Guide: Preparing for and Surviving Disasters with Survival Skills – CERT (Civilian Emergency Response Team) trained and Disaster Recovery Specialist, Richard Lowe, lays out how to make you, your family, and your friends ready for any disaster, large or small. Based upon specialized training, interviews with experts and personal experience, Lowe answers the big question: what is the secret to improving the odds of survival even after a big disaster?

Creating a Bug Out Bag to Save Your Life: What you need to pack for emergency evacuations - When you are ordered to evacuate—or leave of your free will—you probably won't have a lot of time to gather your belongings and the things you'll need. You may have just a few minutes to get out of your home. The best preparation for evacuation is to create what is called a bug out bag. These are also known as go-bags, as in, "grab it and go!"

Professional Freelance Writer Series

How to Operate a Freelance Writing Business, and How to be a Ghostwriter – Proven Tips and Tricks Every Author Needs to Know about Freelance Writing: Insider Secrets from a Professional Ghostwriter – This book explains how to be a ghostwriter, and gives tips on everything from finding customers to creating a statement of work to delivering your final product.

How to Write a Blog That Sells and How to Make Money From Blogging: Insider Secrets from a Professional Blogger: Proven Tips and Tricks Every Blogger Needs to Know to Make Money – There is an art to writing an article that prompts the reader to make a decision to do something. That's the narrow focus of this book. You will learn how to create an article that gets a reader interested, entices them, informs them, and causes them to make a decision when they reach the end.

<u>Other Books by Richard Lowe Jr</u>

<u>How to Be Friends with Women: How to Surround Yourself with Beautiful Women without Being Sleazy</u> – I am a photographer and frequently find myself surrounded by some of the most beautiful women in the world. This book explains how men can attract women and keep them as friends, which can often lead to real, fulfilling relationships.

<u>How to Throw Parties like a Professional: Tips to Help You Succeed with Putting on a Party Event</u> – Many of us have put on parties, and I know it can be a daunting and confusing experience. In this book, I share what I learned from hosting small house parties to shows and events.

Additional Resources

Is your career important to you? Find out how to move your career in any direction you desire, improve your long-term livelihood, and be prepared for any eventuality. Visit the page below to sign up to receive valuable tips via email, and to get a free eBook about how to optimize your LinkedIn profile.

http://list.thewritingking.com/

I've written and published many books on a variety of subjects. They are all listed on the following page.

https://www.thewritingking.com/books/

On that site, I also publish articles about business, writing, and other subjects. You can visit by clicking the following link:

https://www.thewritingking.com

To find out more about me or my photography, you can visit these sites:

Personal website: https://www.richardlowe.com
Photography: http://www.richardlowejr.com
LinkedIn Profile: https://www.linkedin.com/in/richardlowejr
Twitter: https://twitter.com/richardlowejr

If you have any comments about this book, feel free to email me at rich@thewritingking.com

Premium Writing Services

Do you have a story that needs to be told? Have you been trying to write a book for ages but never can seem to find the time to get it done? Do you want to brand your business, but don't know how to get started?

The Writing King has the answer. We can help you with any of your writing needs.

Ghostwriting. We can write your book, which entails interviewing you to get your story, writing the book and then working with you to revise it until complete. To discuss your book, contact The Writing King today.

Website Copy. Many businesses include the text on their sites as an afterthought, and that can result in lost sales and leads. Hire The Writing King to review your site and recommend changes to the text which will help communicate your message and improve your sales.

Blogging. Build engagement with your customers by hiring us to write a weekly or semi-weekly article for your blog, LinkedIn or other social media. Contact The Writing King today to discuss your blogging needs.

LinkedIn. LinkedIn is of the most important vehicles for finding new business, and a professionally written profile works to pulling in those leads. Write or update your profile today.

Technical Writing. We have broad experience in the computer, warehousing and retail industries, and have written hundreds of technical documents. Contact <u>The Writing King</u> today to find out how we can help you with your technical writing project.

<u>The Writing King</u> has the skills and knowledge to help you with any of your writing needs. Call us today to discuss how we can help you.

www.ingramcontent.com/pod-product-compliance
Lightning Source LLC
Chambersburg PA
CBHW071516210326
41597CB00018B/2782